The Diet of Daniel

The Diet of Daniel

a 10 day diet to blessed health, weight loss, and fitness

A practical spiritual guide to eating right, losing weight, getting fit, and staying healthy.

Ernest Edsel

Writers Club Press
San Jose New York Lincoln Shanghai

The Diet of Daniel
a 10 day diet to blessed health, weight loss, and fitness

Writers Club Press
an imprint of iUniverse, Inc.

For information address:
iUniverse, Inc.
5220 S. 16th St., Suite 200
Lincoln, NE 68512
www.iuniverse.com

ISBN: 0-595-21812-1

Printed in the United States of America

To Cristina Zárate Pérez, my beloved mother.

Contents

Foreword

10 DAYS THAT WILL CHANGE YOUR LIFE

This book is a practical spiritual guide to eating right, losing weight, getting fit, and staying healthy.

The book has an introduction and ten chapters. That's one chapter for each of the ten days of the diet.

Every chapter has a bible story to inspire and guide you. And there's a checklist for food and exercise.

After you finish reading the ten chapters, start reading them again. Begin with the first chapter.

Go through the entire cycle of daily readings three times. That will take you through your first month.

Repeat the entire cycle of readings three more times. By then you will have followed the Diet of Daniel for four months. You will then be well on the road to health and fitness.

Don't forget to read Appendix "A" and "B" at the end of the book.

Appendix "A" has a list of recommended supplements, foods, drinks, and exercise. Appendix "B" has a list of scientific sources that prove the Diet of Daniel will bless you with good health.

Appendix "C" is your diet journal. It lets you keep track of your weight and health.

Introduction

WHAT ARE YOU INTERESTED IN?

Are you interested in eating right?

Losing weight?

Getting fit?

Staying healthy?

If you answered yes, then this book is for you. It will help you eat right, lose weight, get fit, and stay healthy.

Few things are more important than your health. Good health lets you enjoy life.

Health and fitness are more than important goals. Good health is essential to a good life. Good health is a blessing. You can't really enjoy your family and loved ones if you are sick in bed. Without good health, you will have a hard time making your dreams come true.

FAITH

Got faith?

You need faith in life. Especially if you're going to do anything that's worthwhile.

Faith is the engine that pulls you to great blessings.

You need faith to get healthy. And stay healthy. You also need faith to lose weight. You really need faith if you're going to be fit.

Lack of faith kept me from getting healthy. I was unhealthy for many years. And very fat. I was totally out-of-shape.

Lack of faith kept me from starting a diet. And when I started a diet, I always quit a few weeks later when I didn't see any results. Loss of faith made me drop out of many diets.

This book will help you keep faith in yourself and your health goals. Faith is what got me to get healthy. And fit. And I lost 200 pounds.

200 POUNDS

It's sad but true. Throughout my childhood and youth, I was very fat and in poor health. I had asthma. If I didn't have a cold or a fever, then I had an ear infection.

I was 200 pounds overweight when I went to medical school. But I lost the 200 pounds in four months. And I kept them off for more than 20 years. I also got healthy and very fit.

THE DIET OF DANIEL

How did I lose 200 pounds? How did I get healthy and fit? I followed the Diet of Daniel.

The diet is ancient. It's time-tested, definitely not a fad.

The diet is from the Bible. It's in the Old Testament.

Here it is:

> *Daniel then said to the guard…"Please test your servants for ten days: Give us nothing but vegetables to eat and water to drink…"*
> *So he agreed to this and tested them for ten days.*
> *At the end of the ten days they looked healthier and better nourished than any of the young men who ate the royal food.*
> —Daniel 1:11-15, *NIV*

DANIEL

Do you remember Daniel?

His life is told in the Book of Daniel. He lived in Israel. He loved God very much. But times were tough. The Assyrians conquered Israel. The new king sent young Daniel as a captive to Babylon in 606 B.C.

Daniel lived in the king's palace. The king's servants tried to feed Daniel. But he refused to eat the refined foods of the palace. Daniel went on a ten day diet. The king's servants worried. They thought Daniel would get sick without the king's rich foods. Daniel proved the diet worked. The diet kept him healthy. He was then able to do great things.

Daniel's diet worked for me. It got me healthy. I lost the 200 pounds. And I've enjoyed many blessings. The diet changed my life.

THE DIET DELIVERS

The Diet of Daniel really delivers. My health and weight are in tiptop shape.

Good health is priceless. It lets you enjoy life's blessings. It helps you overcome life's challenges.

Good health has always helped me. I created a computer product after I dropped out of medical school. The product made a lot of money. Financial disasters then came my way. But I survived them. I was a couch potato. But I now climb 12,000 foot mountains. Good health lets me spend time with family and friends and not with doctors.

MORE THAN JUST A DIET

The Bible is the best guide to good health. After all, the word of God teaches us how to be spiritually fit. The Bible is a practical guide on how to get closer to God. And, as a practical guide, the Bible teaches us how to live right.

Living right.

Doesn't that sound good? That's what God wants for us. To have a more abundant life. Christ said:

"I have come so that people may...enjoy life to the full" (John 10:10, WE).

The Bible shows us two things about diets. First: good health is not just about avoiding certain foods or drinks. Second: dieting is a lifestyle of healthy choices.

HEALTHY CHOICES

Did you get that? Let me repeat. Dieting is a lifestyle of healthy choices.

Daniel's diet and life were all about healthy choices.

- In the beginning, Daniel was in trouble. He was a prisoner. He faced challenges and temptations. But he made the right choices: healthy choices.

- First, Daniel chose to THINK RIGHT. He knew that right thinking was the only way he could survive and prosper in Babylon under a mighty king.

- Second, Daniel chose to EAT RIGHT. He knew that right eating was the only way he could keep his faith and do good works.

- Third, Daniel chose RIGHT ACTIVITIES. He knew that right activities, such as exercise, kept him fit. That way he could serve God.

- In the end, Daniel became a ruler. Kings came to him for advice. He was pure enough to receive revelations from God. Daniel knew that right thinking, right eating, and right activity lead to RIGHT LIVING.

RIGHT LIVING

That's what God wants for you: right living.

You will show me the way of life, granting me the joy of your presence and the pleasures of living with you forever. Psalms 16:11, *NLT.*

Jesus knew all about right living. He said:

"*These things have I spoken unto you, that my joy might remain in you, and that your joy might be full*" John 15:11, *KJV*.

With right living, you break through to blessed health and many other blessings. Just like Daniel.

BREAKING THROUGH

Daniel's diet helped me break free of compulsive overeating. I started eating the right foods. After a lifetime of inactivity, I started exercising. I used to hate exercise, but I soon grew to like it.

More important, Daniel's diet changed my way of thinking. That's the beauty of the Bible, God's word. It changes how you think, how you see yourself. *You are what you think in your heart* (Proverbs 23:7).

When I changed my way of thinking, I changed my behavior. I changed how I saw myself and food. The pounds fell away and stayed away. I got healthier. Nowadays, I'm trim and fit. My resting heart rate is 48 beats per minute. I rarely get sick. I've only seen a doctor two times in twenty-five years.

Would you like to be like Daniel?

Would you like to break through to blessed health and fitness?

If so, follow the Diet of Daniel.

TEN DAY DIET

Here's the Diet of Daniel:

right thinking (day 1 to day 5)

+

right eating (day 6 to day 8)

+

right activity (day 9 to day 10)

=

right living (the rest of your life).

1

RIGHT THINKING

❧

DAY ONE: I WILL HONOR GOD

o o o o o o o o o o o o o o o o o o o o o o o o o o o o o o

You were bought at a price.

Therefore honor God with your body.

——*1 Corinthians 6:20, NIV*

Dieting is about taking care of your body. That is God's commandment. We are literally told to honor God with our body.

If you take care of your body, then you can live at your maximum potential.

How do you care for your body? One way is to eat the foods that Daniel ate.

The king's servant told Daniel that he and his friends had to drink the king's wine and eat the king's rich foods. That was the king's order.

Daniel refused. Instead, he said:

"*...give us pulse to eat, and water to drink*" Daniel 1:12, *KJV*.

What does "pulse" mean?

"Pulse" means a plant that produces seeds. Daniel therefore ate a diet of vegetables, fruits, and grains.

Begin eating Daniel's diet on this first day. Chapter 6 describes the foods in Daniel's diet. See also Chapters 7 and 8. The section called

"Thoughts for Day Eight" in Chapter 8 has a very specific list of healthy foods.

Take a look at Appendix "A" at the end of the book. It has a list of good and bad stuff to eat and drink. Appendix "A" also has the diet supplements that Dr. Andrew Weil, M.D., recommends. He studied at Harvard. And he wrote the national bestseller *Eight Weeks to Optimum Health*.

YOUR CHECKLIST FOR DAY 1

Right Thinking:

I will honor God.   I was bought at a price.   Therefore I will honor God with my body.

Right Eating:

- I will eat the right foods in any amount. I will not go hungry. I will not eat anything with sugar, bread, flour, or red meat. I will eat lots of vegetables. If I must have meat, I will eat fish or fowl (chicken, etc.).

- I will drink plenty of water, alone or in herbal tea. I will only drink pure water.

- I will take a multi-vitamin, multi-mineral supplement. I will also take fresh ginger root, selenium, and other supplements recommended by Dr. Andrew Weil, M.D.

Right Activity:

- I will walk around the block for at least 15 minutes. Or swim. Or do another exercise.

- I will learn what I need to eat and drink. Therefore, I will read the book *Eight Weeks to Optimum Health* by Dr. Andrew Weil, M.D.

I will get this book new or used from a bookstore. Or from the library. Or I will go to the ABalanced Living@ section of **www.drweil.com**.

- I will read the Bible and pray for 15 minutes.

- I will throw away all the bad food in my house. I will throw away all cookies and potato chips. And any other salty, starchy, or sugary snack. I will only snack on fresh vegetables or fruits.

THOUGHTS FOR DAY 1

MODERN DAY DANIELS

Look around. We live in a modern day Babylon. If you're like Daniel, you will want to avoid today's Babylon.

We live in a Babylon of refined foods.

Mounds of food are pushed on us.

Snacks.

Fast food.

Prepared foods.

Few are the foods and drinks that do not have added sugar or salt.

Also, modern society makes us inactive. We become couch potatoes.

Overweight.

Out of shape.

Out of breath.

It's easy to get trapped in the new Babylon: a Babylon of bad health, obesity, poor fitness.

A BABYLON OF FOOD

We live in a Babylon of food.

Want proof?

Consider this: *61% of all Americans are overweight.*

This shocking number comes from the U.S. Surgeon General. It's in the 2001 U.S. Surgeon General Report on Obesity. The report is available in the Surgeon General's website (**www.surgeongeneral. gov/topics/obesity/**).

Consider that: *30% of all Americans are obese.*

Obese isn't just a few extra pounds. It's when a person's weight is more than 20% of their ideal body weight.

Obesity cost $117 billion in 2000. Those were the direct and indirect costs. And that's the bill for just one year!

Remember: 60 million Americans have cardiovascular disease. Heart disease makes up 40% of all deaths.

Think about this: more than 13 million Americans suffer from adult-onset diabetes.

Diabetes is nasty. You've seen the ugly symptoms. Exhaustion. Mood swings. Overeating.

Diabetes destroys many organs. Like kidneys. And eyes. Circulation gets bad in the arms and legs. Amputations are sometimes necessary. That's why it's so important to control diabetes with diet.

TIME FOR ACTION

I was very fat and in bad health. But I was comfortable in my situation. I just didn't care. My weight had ballooned after gorging on dorm food in college. Afterwards, I was too busy studying in med school. All that changed one evening.

Our anatomy professor was talking about the three body types that the ancient Greeks had observed. He called two of my friends to the front of the class.

Maurice was the first one to be called. He was a perfect example of ectoderm: tall, skinny, and nervous.

The class giggled.

David was next. He was a perfect example of mesoderm: muscular, slow, and powerful.

Laughter broke out. David blushed.

The professor looked around the class. He said:

"Endoderm. The Greeks thought that the endoderm was obese, good-natured, and lazy."

The professor called me. My heart sank as I walked to the front of the room. The class howled with laughter.

I went home that night. Angry. Hurt. More than anything, I was devastated at the thought that I was part of a freak show. An object of laughter.

I realized two things.

First, I was 100% responsible for my situation. I had gotten careless. Let myself go. I knew I was bloated. It had been a year since I had weighed myself at 330 pounds. And I had kept overeating that whole year! I rarely found clothes that fit me. My mother had to cut open my pants and add fabric.

Second, I realized I was a hypocrite. How could I become a doctor when I was fat and in bad health?

I decided to change. To lose weight. To eat right. To get healthy.

I threw away every bag of snacks in my apartment. I stopped buying bad foods. No more cookies or bread. I stopped eating unhealthy foods. No more pizza. No more fast food.

A good friend, Edward, took me walking every morning. Soon I was running with his father, Dr. Fortin Garcia. He ran up a hill every day. He was an anesthesiologist. Dr. Garcia picked me up every single morning at 4:00 A.M. I lost 200 pounds in less than four months.

I read the Bible every day. And prayed. The Book of Daniel inspired me. Like Daniel, I made up my mind to get healthy. And health came to me.

2

RIGHT THINKING

❖

DAY TWO: I WILL START RIGHT WITH RIGHT THINKING

o o o o o o o o o o o o o o o o o o o o o o o o o o o o o o o o

Be strong and of a good courage.

——*Joshua 1:6, KJV*

You started Daniel's diet.

But how are you going to keep the diet?

Only one way: right thinking.

Right thinking gets you motivated. It lets you focus. Stay on course. The old saying is true: it takes guts to start a diet. It takes even more guts to keep a diet.

Daniel had to get motivated. He was in a very difficult situation. His family and friends had expectations about him. They expected him to stand firm in his faith while he lived in pagan Babylon.

Babylon has tested the faith of men and women throughout history.

Sodom and Gomorrah were immoral. But Babylon was the worst because of her wealth and power. She's mentioned time and again in the Old and New Testament.

The prophet Jeremiah lived at the time of Daniel. They probably knew each other.

Jeremiah wrote this about Babylon:

Babylon…made the whole earth drunk. The nations drank her wine; therefore they have now gone mad (Jeremiah 51:7, *NIV*).

John the Revelator wrote:

The great city of Babylon…This is the city that made all nations drunk and immoral (Revelation 14:8, *CEV*).

We face a Babylon of fattening and unhealthy foods. But we can take a stand and win, just like Daniel.

You can do it. Be like Daniel. The good thing is that no one will beat, jail, or kill you if you refuse to eat unhealthy food. Daniel, on the other hand, was in personal danger when he went on a diet.

Why?

Because Daniel was disobeying the king by going on a diet. That was dangerous. Kings often killed, jailed, or tortured their subjects, especially the disobedient.

Daniel was in a lot of danger when he rejected the king's wines and rich foods. The king's servant told Daniel:

"The king has decided what you must eat and drink. And I am afraid he will kill me, if you eat something else and end up looking worse than the other young men" (Daniel 1:10, *CEV*).

Like Daniel, you're under pressure or stress. At home or work. Sure, they're different stresses than the ones Daniel had. But stress is part of the human condition. That's why right thinking is so important.

YOUR CHECKLIST FOR DAY 2

Right Thinking:

I am strong and have good courage. I have the courage to start the Diet of Daniel. I am strong enough to keep the diet.

Right Eating:

- I eat the right foods in any amount. I will not go hungry. I will not eat anything with sugar, bread, flour, or red meat. I will eat lots of vegetables. If I must have meat, I will eat fish or fowl (chicken, etc.).

- I drink plenty of water, alone or in herbal tea. I only drink pure water.

- I take a multi-vitamin, multi-mineral supplement. I also take fresh ginger root, selenium, and other supplements recommended by Dr. Andrew Weil, M.D.

Right Activity:

- I walk around the block for at least 15 minutes. Or swim. Or do another exercise.

- I read the Bible and pray for 15 minutes.

- I only snack on fresh vegetables or fruits.

THOUGHTS FOR DAY 2

DANIEL IN BABYLON

Imagine life in 606 B.C. That was more than 2,600 years ago. Back then, Babylon was a rich city.

Powerful.

Beautiful.

The city rose out of the hot, fertile plains of Iraq. The great river Euphrates flowed past the city. The famous hanging gardens of Babylon crowned the city.

Babylon was the center of government. Like Washington, D.C. It was also a hothouse of culture. And a financial powerhouse. Think of

New York City. Last, but not least, a city of sin: think Las Vegas. Imagine all those cities rolled into one.

The city was meant to impress.

Seduce.

Overwhelm.

Modern society is like Babylon.

Advertising is meant to impress us. To convince us. To brainwash us. That's why food companies spend so much money on advertising.

Guess how much companies spend in advertising food and drinks to you and me?

Fifty billion dollars.

They tell us to buy and eat all sorts of foods. Especially unhealthy foods. And fattening foods. You know their names: fast food and junk food. And McDonald's. And Burger King. And Wendy's.

We are constantly bombarded with advertising for food. Cookies. Crackers. Bread. Pizza. Snacks.

Advertising also tells us to drink all sorts of beverages loaded with sugar or caffeine.

Movies seduce us. We're told to drink booze. Smoke. Do drugs. You name it.

Gadgets lure us into inactivity. We don't exercise. We drive our cars everywhere. We watch too much television. And our children play all day long with video games and computer games.

Daniel overcame Babylon with his diet. So can you. Just follow the diet.

MUST HAVE SUPPLEMENTS

Make sure you take the supplements recommended by Dr. Weil. The supplements boost the benefits of Daniel's diet. Dr. Weil should know. He studied medicine at Harvard.

I read his book (*8 Weeks to Optimum Health*). It greatly improved my life. I take all the supplements he recommends (vitamins, minerals, ginger, and selenium).

I rarely get a cold or the flu. And when I do, they're mild and quickly go away. See Appendix "A" at the end of the book. It has a list of the supplements recommended by Dr. Weil.

3

RIGHT THINKING

❖

DAY THREE: WATCH AND PRAY

o o o o o o o o o o o o o o o o o o o o o o o o o o o o o o
Watch and pray so that you   will not fall into temptation.
  The spirit is willing,   but the body is weak.
——*Matthew 26:41, NIV*

God has a diet for you. That diet is Daniel's diet. But the road to health and fitness has challenges. Every great journey has challenges.

You will face two challenges on the road to health and fitness.

The first challenge: discouragement, or lack of motivation.

The second challenge: temptations, lots of them.

Early in my life, I met discouragement and temptation. Thanks to them I was 200 pounds overweight. But I lost the 200 pounds. And I kept them off for more than 20 years.

I lost the weight because I got motivated. I knew that if I followed the diet, then I would get the results I wanted. So, I followed the Diet of Daniel. I also got motivated by reading the Bible. And praying.

Trust me, I was tempted with hunger that first week. Cravings hunted me. But I never once caved in. I just ate more healthy foods. Whenever I was hungry, I ate the right foods. And I did more exercise.

Don't think you won't be tempted. Jesus was tempted by hunger. Bread was the first temptation offered to a hungry Jesus!

Jesus went on a fast. He had no food for 40 days and nights (Matthew 4:2). Satan asked Jesus to turn a stone into bread (Matthew 4:3). But Jesus refused to make the stone into bread. Instead, Jesus said:

"No one can live only on food. People need every word that God has spoken" (Matthew 4:3, *CEV*).

It's true: you do not live by bread alone.

Everyone suffers from temptation. After you overcome temptation, you do great things. That's how life worked out for Jesus. First, He was tempted in the desert. He rejected temptation. Then He went on his divine mission. It'll be the same way for you. First, you will be tempted when you're on the diet. You will reject temptation. Then you will be healthy and fit.

Your mission is to be healthy and fit!

So watch yourself and pray. Then you will be blessed with good health and fitness. Don't just live on food. Feast on the word of God.

YOUR CHECKLIST FOR DAY 3

Right Thinking:

I watch and pray so I do not fall into temptation. I keep my diet. I am headed to the Promised Land of health and fitness.

Right Eating:

- I'm eating the right foods. I never go hungry. I never eat anything with sugar, bread, flour, or red meat. I'm eating lots of vegetables. If I must have meat, I eat fish or fowl (chicken, etc.).

- I'm drinking plenty of water, alone or in herbal tea. I'm only drinking pure water.

- I'm taking a multi-vitamin, multi-mineral supplement. I'm also taking fresh ginger root, selenium, and other supplements recommended by Dr. Andrew Weil, M.D.

Right Activity:

- I walk around the block for at least 15 minutes. Or swim. Or do another exercise.

- I'm reading the Bible and pray for 15 minutes.

- I'm only snacking on fresh vegetables or fruits.

THOUGHTS FOR DAY 3

MOSES

Every worthwhile journey has challenges. Your journey to good health will have challenges.

Moses faced many challenges when he led his people out of Egypt. They easily got discouraged. That's why they complained about how much they missed the flesh pots of Egypt: *"when we did eat bread to the full"* (Exodus 16:3, *KJV*).

Moses led the twelve tribes of Israel out of slavery. But Pharaoh fed his slaves well. Food had a very strong hold over the twelve tribes of Israel. They missed the foods of slavery when they went out into the desert with Moses. The people accused Moses: *for ye have brought us forth into this wilderness, to kill this whole assembly with hunger* (Numbers 11:18, *KJV*).

Many folks prefer to be slaves to the Pharaoh of salt, sugar, starch, and fat. I've been a prisoner in the kingdom of cookies, pizza, snacks, fast food, and junk food. But I broke free. So can you.

You're not a slave. That's why you're stepping out to freedom. You're on your way to the Promised Land of health and fitness. Sure, you'll be tempted. But you won't quit.

The Diet of Daniel will bless you.

4

RIGHT THINKING

✦

DAY FOUR: THE POWER OF ONE

o o o o o o o o o o o o o o o o o o o o o o o o o o o o o o o

Don't be afraid, for I am with you.
 Do not be dismayed, for I am your God.
 I will strengthen you. I will help you.
 I will uphold you with my victorious right hand.
—*Isaiah 41:10, NLT*

Babylon was powerful. She was the capital of an empire: the Assyrian empire. The great empire grew by war. It conquered Israel. The prophet Jeremiah wrote that God made Babylon supreme:

This is what the LORD Almighty, the God of Israel, says: I will put an iron yoke on the necks of all these nations to make them serve Nebuchadnezzar king of Babylon, and they will serve him. I will even give him control over the wild animals.
—Jeremiah 28:14, *NIV*

So, imagine how imposing Babylon was to a young man like Daniel. He came from Israel. Back then, Israel was a small nothing of a country. Defeated in war, Israel was broken, a subject nation.

Daniel could have felt he was a nobody.

Weak.

Powerless.

Conquered.

But Daniel did not feel that way. Not even when he faced King Nebuchadnezzar.

The mighty king had a subtle plan for Daniel. Nebuchadnezzar ordered his court to teach the best of the young men he had captured in Israel. The king wanted to train Daniel and three other young men from Israel. They were to become part of the king's government.

The king was smart. He expected Daniel to give up his faith after Daniel was exposed to the religion of a great military power. But Daniel had a better plan: his diet.

Daniel's diet made him powerful. He resisted the king's subtle plan. By keeping his diet, Daniel kept his faith. God therefore blessed Daniel.

The king made Daniel a ruler. Daniel became "*chief of the governors*" (Daniel 2:48).

Why?

Because Daniel had faith to keep the diet. Daniel showed courage and integrity. The diet also made Daniel the best he could be.

Daniel's three friends followed his diet. They were blessed. The king gave them important jobs in his government (Daniel 2:49).

The Bible is clear about the blessings of the diet. God gave the four young men knowledge and skill…In addition, he gave Daniel skill in interpreting visions and dreams.

At the end of the three years…The king talked with them all, and Daniel…[and his three friends]…impressed him more than any of the others.

So they became members of the king's court. No matter what question the king asked or what problem he raised, these four knew ten times more than any fortuneteller or magician in his whole kingdom.

——Daniel 1:17-20, *GNT*

The Diet of Daniel will bless you. Your mind will be clear. Your body will be healthy. More blessings will come your way.

YOUR CHECKLIST FOR DAY 4

Right Thinking:

God is with me. I am not afraid. He will strengthen me. He will help me.

Right Eating:

- I eat the right foods in any amount. I will not go hungry. I will not eat anything with sugar, bread, flour, or red meat. I will eat lots of vegetables. If I must have meat, I will eat fish or fowl (chicken, etc.).

- I drink plenty of water, alone or in herbal tea. I only drink pure water.

- I take a multi-vitamin, multi-mineral supplement. I also take fresh ginger root, selenium, and other supplements recommended by Dr. Andrew Weil, M.D.

Right Activity:

- I walk around the block for at least 20 minutes. Or swim. Or do another exercise.

- I read the Bible and pray for 15 minutes.

- I only snack on fresh vegetables or fruits.

THOUGHTS FOR DAY 4

IN THE IMAGE OF GOD

Nebuchadnezzar wanted the best and brightest to work for him. That's why the king picked the children of the nobility of his newest conquests. Daniel was one of them. You're like Daniel. You are also of noble blood. *You are the child of a most high God* (Psalm 82:6, *NLT*).

Remember: you are made in God's image. *So God created human beings, making them to be like himself. He created them male and female* (Genesis 1:27, *GNT*).

Like Daniel and his three friends, you can keep yourself from falling under the influence of today's Babylon: a Babylon of unhealthy foods and physical inactivity.

Keep your heavenly image. How? By keeping the Diet of Daniel. Keep it no matter how many more times you're challenged. You can do it. I did. Daniel and his three friends did.

KEEP THE FAITH

God blessed Daniel. And his three friends.

How?

They got powerful jobs.

But Daniel's friends were tested again. The King wanted them to give up their faith. He told them to worship an image of gold (Daniel 3:1). The three men refused. The king gave an order: the men were to be thrown into a fire (Daniel 3:12-25).

Did they die?

No. They survived without a single burn! God protected them. See, Daniel 3:26-27.

Why did Daniel's friends survive?

Because they were prepared: physically and spiritually.

How?

With the Diet of Daniel. The diet purified and strengthened them.

The king was amazed. He promoted them. He also ordered that the three men were never to be harmed (Daniel 3:29-30).

IN THE LIONS' DEN

Daniel was tested again.

Nebuchadnezzar died. His son became the new king. He threw a big party. His guests drank lots of wine. The new king used the gold and silver cups that his father had captured from the Temple (Daniel 5:1-4).

A strange writing appeared on a wall during the party (Daniel 5:5). The writing troubled the king. Daniel read the writing. He understood it. Daniel told the king that his kingdom would end (Daniel 5:25-28).

Daniel's prophesy came true the night he said it. That's how powerful the diet had made Daniel. He had become a pure instrument of God.

Darius conquered Babylon on that fateful night. He was the king of Persia (Iran).

Darius made Daniel the highest of all princes in Babylon (Daniel 6). The other princes grew jealous of Daniel. They convinced the king to pass a new law. The law prohibited anyone from worshiping God. But Daniel kept his faith: he prayed and worshiped God.

The king liked Daniel. But he had to punish Daniel. Daniel had blatantly disobeyed the king's order. So Daniel was thrown into a den of lions.

The following morning the king ran to the den. He was sure that the lions had ripped Daniel to pieces. But Daniel was alive. Unharmed.

Keep the Diet of Daniel. You will walk out of many lions' dens unharmed. The diet will give you the strength of good health.

MY OWN EXPERIENCE

Fate threw me into many lions' dens. But I always walked away unharmed.

Why?

Because I keep the diet.

In 1995, I lost a small fortune in bad investments. I then moved to Portland, Oregon. I had less than $200 in my pocket. I immediately found a good job. And partly rebuilt my wealth.

Two years later, I injured my neck. I had horrible headaches. And muscle spasms in my neck. My right hand broke out with eczema. But I instantly recovered. All I needed: one chiropractic treatment.

The doctor told me I was the exception. He said: "Most of my patients don't recover so quickly. They don't eat right or exercise."

That's the power of the Diet of Daniel. It keeps you going even after you get hurt or sick. It protects you when you're in the lions' dens.

5

RIGHT THINKING

*

DAY FIVE: THE VALUE OF APPRECIATION

o o o o o o o o o o o o o o o o o o o o o o o o o o o o
You have shown me the path to life, and you make me glad
by being near to me. Sitting at your right side, I will always
be joyful.
—*Psalms 16:11, CEV*

The Bible shows you the path to life. The Diet of Daniel is the path
to a healthy life. It's easy to keep the diet if you value good health
and fitness.

I appreciate good health. But I really value good health when I get
sick. Like the time I injured my neck. That's when I really valued good
health.

Some people are naturally blessed with good health. But many of
them take it for granted. Do you take good health for granted? Or do
you want it badly?

If we don't appreciate good health, we become like Esau. He did not
value his birthright.

A BOWL OF FOOD

As the firstborn of Isaac, Esau had a birthright. He was going to inherit everything his father owned. Isaac was very wealthy. He had everything. Servants. Flocks. Herds. But Esau lost everything because he did not value his birthright. He traded it for a bowl of pottage (lentils). Esau had another problem. He simply could not control his appetite (Genesis 25: 29-34).

Are you like Esau? Or are you like Jacob?

Jacob valued Esau's birthright. Jacob offered his brother the bowl of food. In return, he got Esau's inheritance. That's why Jacob became the patriarch of a nation with his twelve sons (Genesis 35: 11, 22).

So do you really value health and fitness?

I think you do.

You know what good health does for you. Good health lets you care for yourself and your family.

Pay bills.

Get and hold a job.

Succeed in a career.

Raise a family.

Get closer to God.

Claim your birthright. Claim your inheritance. Claim good health. Just do it: keep the Diet of Daniel.

YOUR CHECKLIST FOR DAY 5

Right Thinking:

God shows me the path to life. God makes me glad by being near to me. I sit at the right side of God. I claim my inheritance of good health.

Right Eating:

- I eat the right foods in any amount. I will not go hungry. I will not eat anything with sugar, bread, flour, or red meat. I eat lots of vegetables. If I must have meat, I eat fish or fowl (chicken, etc.).

- I drink plenty of water, alone or in herbal tea. I only drink pure water.

- I take a multi-vitamin, multi-mineral supplement. I also take fresh ginger root, selenium, and other supplements recommended by Dr. Andrew Weil, M.D.

Right Activity:

- I walk around the block for at least 20 minutes. Or swim. Or do another exercise.

- I read the Bible and pray for 15 minutes.

- I only snack on fresh vegetables or fruits.

THOUGHTS FOR DAY 5

STORY OF VERONICA

Good health was very important to Jesus Christ. Sick people mobbed Him. They desperately wanted miracle cures. The crowds were huge. A paralyzed man had to be lowered through a roof so Jesus could heal him (Mark 2:4).

A woman called Veronica wanted to be healed. She had been sick for 12 years. She pushed her way through the crowd. She only wanted to touch Jesus's coat (Luke 8:43-44). She was immediately healed when she touched His coat.

Veronica was desperate. She had spent her fortune on doctors (Luke 8:43). They did nothing for her. Her health came back when she reached out to Jesus and claimed good health. So can you if you are in bad health. Claim good health. Act on it. Reach out and keep the diet.

Poor health will empty your bank account. Just like Veronica.

Bad health is emptying our bank accounts. We spend billions of dollars on healthcare.

How many dollars?

$146 billion. That's what we spent on the medical services industry. Stuff like doctor visits. And surgery. Or lab tests. And that was just for calendar year 2000. Isn't that incredible? It's sad but true. This information comes from Value Line, a respected financial publisher.

Keep the Diet of Daniel and you will save a fortune. And save yourself.

STORY OF JOB

Most people <u>say</u> they want good health and fitness. But very few people do anything about it. A very small minority keeps a lifetime diet or exercise program.

Bad health affects your body and your purse. And your mind. And soul. Poor health drags you down mentally and spiritually.

Satan knows how important good health is to us. Satan uses bad health to attack and weaken us. Bad health can break you down. Just ask Job.

Do you remember Job?

He was extremely faithful. Even after he was tested by Satan.

How did Satan test Job's faith?

Satan got him sick (Job 2:6-7).

Satan planned to destroy Job's faith with bad health. Job had already lost his fortune and children. But Job had kept his faith. That's why Satan threw a skin disease at Job. Satan expected to crush Job with bad health.

So Job came down with painful boils. His faith was sorely tested. Job's wife told him to curse God and die (Job 2:9). But he did not. Instead he said:

"Shall we accept good from God, and not trouble?" (Job 2:10, *NIV*).

Appreciate good health. It has great value. If you appreciate good health, then you will be able to keep the Diet of Daniel.

6

RIGHT EATING

✦

DAY SIX: GOD'S FOOD

o o o o o o o o o o o o o o o o o o o o o o o o o o o o o o o o o

"…you will eat the plants of the field."

——*Genesis 3:18, NIV*

Dieting is not about denying yourself great foods. Dieting is not about starving to death. Dieting is all about eating right. It's about enjoying all the good food that God put on this earth.

In Genesis 1:29, *NIV*, God said:

"I give you every seed-bearing plant on the face of the whole earth and every tree that has fruit with seed in it. They will be yours for food." The Bible is clear: God wants us to eat vegetables, grains, and fruit. That's the Diet of Daniel.

Do you remember that Daniel asked for pulse? See Daniel 1:12. Pulse means a plant that produces seeds. Daniel therefore ate a diet of vegetables, fruits, and grains. That's God's diet.

Let me repeat: God told us to eat vegetables, grains, and fruit. They are seed-bearing plants. God gave this diet to Adam and Eve in the Garden of Eden (Genesis 1:29).

After Adam and Eve left Eden, God again told them to keep the vegetarian diet. God said:

"you will eat the plants of the field" (Genesis 3:18, *NIV*).

People lived for a long time when they followed God's diet. Adam lived until he was 930 years old. From Adam to Noah, people got to be very old.

How old?

More than 500 years old!

Scientific studies prove that the Diet of Daniel works. That's what the American Heart Association and others say. See Appendix "B" at the end of the book. It lists the scientific sources that prove the Diet of Daniel will bless you with good health.

It's true. If you cut back on meat, you will be healthier. You'll have a lower risk of getting cancer. Ditto for heart disease. And you're less likely to have a degenerative disease like arthritis.

The Diet of Daniel will bless you with good health. That's a scientific fact.

YOUR CHECKLIST FOR DAY 6

Right Thinking:

God gave me a diet. He first gave it to Adam and Eve in the Garden of Eden. Daniel kept God's diet. So will I. I will eat plants and fruits, just as God commands.

Right Eating:

- I eat the right foods in any amount. I will not go hungry. I will not eat anything with sugar, bread, flour, or red meat. I eat lots of vegetables. If I must have meat, I eat fish or fowl (chicken, etc.).

- I drink plenty of water, alone or in herbal tea. I only drink pure water.

- I take a multi-vitamin, multi-mineral supplement. I also take fresh ginger root, selenium, and other supplements recommended by Dr. Andrew Weil, M.D.

Right Activity:

- I walk around the block for at least 20 minutes. Or swim. Or do another exercise.

- I will learn more about what I need to eat and drink.

  Therefore, I will read the book "The Pritikin Weight Loss Breakthrough" by Robert Pritikin.

  I will get this book new or used from a bookstore. Or from the library.

- I read the Bible and pray for 15 minutes.

- I only snack on fresh vegetables or fruits.

THOUGHTS FOR DAY 6

GOD'S FOOD IS NOT BORING.

God's food tastes great. That's why I love the Diet of Daniel. I eat plenty of raw vegetables, fruits, and grains. I almost never eat any meat. And when I do, I only have seafood or chicken.

So what do I eat every day?

Three cups of raw oats. One sliced apple. Lots of prunes. And one or two cups of yogurt.

I also drink plenty of mineral water and soy milk. But not everybody likes raw food. You can steam or boil vegetables and fruits. Or grill the vegetables. Add the right spices. Sprinkle salt, pepper, and oregano on steamed vegetables. Try cinnamon on fruit or oatmeal.

Use lots of spices and herbs. Which ones?

Basil. Cayenne. Chives. Cilantro. Dill. Garlic. Ginger. Oregano. Paprika. Any pepper. Rosemary. Sage. Tarragon. Thyme.

There are a thousand ways to cook vegetables, fruits, and grains. Just look at all the new healthy food cookbooks in your bookstore or library.

The food in Daniel's diet tastes great.

There's no excuse for wanting junk food or fast food.

YOU WILL NEVER GO HUNGRY WITH THIS DIET

All foods in the Diet of Daniel are filling. Very filling. You will not be hungry after you eat Daniel's foods.

Why?

Because they're full of fiber. And high in protein.

I'm never hungry with Daniel's foods. There's lots of fiber and bulk in oats, apples, prunes, and yogurt. I feel very full when that thick combination hits my stomach. I have one huge serving of the combination every day. That's my dinner.

Do I eat anything else in addition to my dinner? You bet. But only if and when I'm hungry. Sometimes I have a vegetable salad. But I usually just have oats and yogurt. Those are my snacks.

I also drink soy milk. There's a great brand called Silk soy milk. It's made by White Wave. Talk about delicious. It has no saturated fats (which are bad for the heart). I have 1 or 2 cups of soy milk after I exercise. It gives me a lot of energy. I usually thicken the soy milk with a high quality soy protein powder. It makes a delicious milkshake.

Don't drink more than 2 cups of soy milk. Or you will get fat. Especially if you're not exercising a lot.

Why?

Because soy milk has sugar, just like cow milk.

YOU WILL ALWAYS BE HUNGRY WITH JUNK FOOD AND FAST FOOD

It's true. Junk food and fast food will NEVER fill you up. The same goes for processed foods. That includes: bread; cookies; crackers; snacks; and, any prepared meal you buy at the supermarket.

Junk food, fast food, and processed foods have no real bulk. And little or no fiber. You will get very hungry thanks to their very high content of fat and carbohydrate (sugar).

Just ask Dr. Rachael Heller. And Dr. Richard Heller. They are medical scientists. They wrote a bestseller: *The Carbohydrate Addict's Diet.* It explains why people get hungry with junk food, fast food, and processed food.

Junk food, fast food, and processed foods never filled me up. They always left me hungry. Very hungry. I constantly overate.

I still remember how hungry I felt after gorging. I used to eat a big bag of "Chips Ahoy!" chocolate chip cookies. And I'd wash them down with a gallon of milk.

Guess what?

Thirty minutes later, I was hungry!

There's no doubt about it. People overeat because they eat junk food, fast food, and processed foods.

7

RIGHT EATING

❦

DAY SEVEN: FROM ADAM TO NOAH TO MOSES

○ ○
But those who trust the LORD will find new strength. They will be strong like eagles soaring upward on wings; they will walk and run without getting tired.
—*Isaiah 40:31, CEV*

Trust the Lord. Eat vegetables, fruits and grains.

Adam trusted the Lord. He ate the foods of the Diet of Daniel. That's why Adam got to be 930 years old (Genesis 5:5).

But then came the Great Flood.

The ark saved Noah, his family, and the animals. People started eating meat. It's not clear why they did this. Maybe they ate some of the animals in the ark.

Why?

Because all vegetables, fruits, and grains died in the flood. It would take time for plants to grow after the flood. One thing is clear. God let humans eat some meat after the flood.

"Every moving thing that lives shall be food for you. I have given you all things, even as the green herbs."
——Gen 9:3, *NKJV*

So people began eating meat.

Guess what happened?

People's lives got shorter.

Moses only lived to be 120 years old.

If you eat meat, your life will be shorter. That's why most people do not live to be 120 years old. Meat is not good for you. See the scientific studies listed in Appendix "B".

On the other hand, you will find new strength if you trust the Lord with the Diet of Daniel. If you eat Daniel's food, you will be as strong as an eagle soaring upward on wings.

Isaiah's promise is true: you will walk and run without getting tired. Follow the Diet of Daniel. Be like Adam and Eve. You will live to a healthy old age.

YOUR CHECKLIST FOR DAY 7

Right Thinking:

I trust God's diet. I find new strength. I am strong. I walk and run without getting tired.

Right Eating:

- I eat the right foods in any amount. I do not go hungry. I do not eat anything with sugar, bread, flour, or red meat. I eat lots of vegetables. I cut back on beef and pork. I never eat them more than once or twice a week. If I must have meat, I eat fish or fowl (chicken, turkey, etc.).

- I drink plenty of water, alone or in herbal tea. I only drink pure water.

- I take a multi-vitamin, multi-mineral supplement. I also take fresh ginger root, selenium, and other supplements recommended by Dr. Andrew Weil, M.D.

Right Activity:

- I walk around the block for at least 25 minutes. Or swim. Or do another exercise.

- I only snack on fresh vegetables or fruits.

- I read the Bible and pray for 15 minutes.

THOUGHTS FOR DAY 7

DIET LAWS OF MOSES

Moses wrote down God's laws and rules for food and diet. They are called "kosher" laws or rules. But almost nobody follows kosher laws about food.

The most important of the kosher laws is where God said: *you must not eat any meat that still has blood in it* (Genesis 9:4, *CEV*).

The law is simple: all blood must be drained out of the animal when the butcher kills the animal.

Do you eat kosher meat? Kosher beef? Kosher chicken?

Probably not. Most people don't.

So if you're going to eat meat, then try to eat kosher meat. It's healthier than regular meat. Kosher food is clearly labeled as "kosher".

THREE MORE RULES

Here are three more kosher laws or rules from Moses.

First: we must not eat animal fat (Leviticus 3:17). But almost all junk food, fast food, and processed food has animal fat.

Second: we must not eat pig meat (Deuteronomy 14:7-8). But almost everybody eats pork. In hot dogs. Bacon. Or pork chops.

Third: we must not eat animals that eat dead flesh. The Bible is very strict about this rule. See, Exodus 22:31; Leviticus 7:24; Leviticus 11:9-10; Deuteronomy 14:9 and 12-16.

But guess what animals eat dead flesh?

Crab. Lobster. And other shellfish.

Pigs too.

It's no big secret: most of us eat lobster, pigs, and other animals that eat dead flesh.

What does this all mean?

It's almost impossible for fast food, junk food, and processed food to meet God's rules.

SAD BUT TRUE

Almost all of our meat now comes from animals that eat dead flesh.

It's sad but true.

Animal feed companies are crazy. First, they buy large amounts of dead sheep, pigs, and cows. Then they mill and mix the dead animal parts into corn, oats, and other grain. This strange feed is then fed to cows, sheep, and pigs.

Guess what?

That's how mad cow disease got into the beef supply and into humans in Europe.

NOT THE SAME

Today's meat is <u>not</u> like the meat from the days of Noah, Moses, and Jesus.

Back then, animals were raised in small herds. They roamed freely. They ate pure, natural foods. Meat was fresh.

That's not the case today.

Animals are now raised in huge numbers. In crowded spaces. It's unhealthy. That's why their feed is laced with antibiotics.

Owners also give hormones and other junk to their animals.

Meat isn't fresh. It usually takes weeks or months for any meat to reach your table. That's not fresh meat. Fresh is a few hours old. Or a day or two at the most.

Cut back on eating meat. Better yet, avoid it. Or eat it once in a blue moon.

8

RIGHT EATING

✦

DAY EIGHT: TEMPLE AND SPIRIT

○ ○
You surely know that your body is a temple where the Holy
Spirit lives. The Spirit is in you and is a gift from God.
—*1 Corinthians 6:19, CEV*

God cares a lot about your health and fitness.

Why?

Because He gave you a temple. Not a shack. But a temple. That temple is your body.

Temples are always built with the best materials. King Solomon built the first temple. He built it with the best stone and wood. Expensive cedar covered every room. The wood was then covered with gold. See, 1 Kings 6:1, 15, and 21.

Are you building your temple with the best materials? What foods do you build your temple with? Good, wholesome food? Or junk food?

Be like Solomon. Build your temple with the best food. Eat lots of vegetables. And fruits. And grains.

Temples are treated with reverence. That's why you must treat your temple with respect.

How?

By keeping in shape. And never letting your temple fall apart with overeating or inactivity.

If you take care of your temple, then God's glory will fill you. That's what happened to the temple when Solomon finished building:

"the glory of the LORD filled his temple" (1 Kings 8:11, *NIV*)

If you build your temple with the best food, then God's glory will fill you. Just like Solomon's temple.

YOUR CHECKLIST FOR DAY 8

Right Thinking:

My body is a temple where the Holy Spirit lives. The Spirit is in me. It is a gift from God. I take good care of my temple.

Right Eating:

- I only eat the best foods: the right foods. I do not go hungry. That's why I eat any amount of the right food. I do not eat anything with sugar, bread, flour, or red meat. I eat lots of vegetables. If I must have meat, I eat fish or fowl (chicken, etc.).

- I will drink plenty of water, alone or in herbal tea. I will only drink pure water.

- I will take a multi-vitamin, multi-mineral supplement. I will also take fresh ginger root, selenium, and other supplements recommended by Dr. Andrew Weil, M.D.

Right Activity:

- I walk around the block for at least 25 minutes. Or swim. Or do another exercise.

- I will read the Bible and pray for 15 minutes.

- I will only snack on fresh vegetables or fruits.

THOUGHTS FOR DAY 8

QUALITY IS THE KEY

Don't worry about how much you're eating with the Diet of Daniel. Instead, look at **_what_** you're eating.

Quality is what counts, not quantity. That's why you will never go hungry if you eat the right food.

Quality counts. That's why Solomon built a great temple with the best materials. You can build your own great temple of a body with the best foods.

Here are some super-healthy foods. They are the best food to eat. Especially if they're organic (with no pesticides).

You can eat several big salads made with:

any leafy vegetable (arugula, endive, romaine, spinach, etc.)

artichoke

asparagus

avocado

beans (black, green, string, snow pea pods, wax, etc.)

beet

bok choy

broccoli

brussel sprouts

cabbage

cauliflower

celery

chard

cucumber

eggplant

greens (collard, dandelion, any leafy green)

heart of palm

jicama

kale

kohlrabi

leek

mushrooms and morels

okra

olives (any)

onion (any)

peppers (any)

pumpkin

rabe

radicchio

radishes

rhubarb

sauerkraut

scallions

shoots or sprouts (bamboo shoots, bean sprouts, etc.)

spinach

squash (spaghetti squash, etc.)

tomato

turnip

water chestnuts

zucchini

So eat salads. Lots of them. You can eat HUGE quantities of leafy or water-filled vegetables (such as carrots, celery, and any lettuce). They have very few calories. They're packed with vitamins and nutrients.

Don't forget to add spices and herbs. Use some olive oil and vinegar. Or lemon juice. Stay away from salad dressings. They usually have sugar and other carbohydrates.

Fruits have natural sugars. Therefore, avoid drinking more than three or four glasses of juice.

Why?

Because juice won't fill you. Instead, eat the actual fruit. It will make you feel full. Also, stay away from juice concentrates. They're loaded with sugar.

If you're a diabetic, make sure you stay within your calorie limits.

PRACTICAL TIPS

Get some "Ziploc" plastic bags. Use them to carry the right food with you at all times. That way you can eat whenever you're hungry. Pack the bags with a salad of celery, carrots, and lettuce. Pack ten bags if that's what you need to prevent hunger at work or home.

Use small tupperware bowls at home or work to microwave and cook foods at LOW HEAT. That way you use the food's natural steam. Or use a little olive oil or margarine.

9

RIGHT ACTIVITY

✦

DAY NINE: FAITH AND WORKS

o o o o o o o o o o o o o o o o o o o o o o o o o o o o o o

Faith without works is dead.

—*James 2:26, NKJV*

F aith plus works equals great results. Just look at Paul the Apostle.

Paul knew a lot about right activity. He built up Christianity. He did this right after Jesus died. Back then, very few people believed in Jesus. But Paul had a vision of Jesus Christ. He accepted Jesus as Lord.

Did Paul then sit at home and just hope for the best?

No. He took action. The right action: physical action.

What physical action?

He walked. And he preached. He went all over Europe. And the Middle East. It wasn't easy. He suffered persecution. Ridicule. Hardship. But he won in the end. He overcame great odds.

Paul's activity paid off. He changed people's lives. He changed history itself. Christianity is now a major religion.

Like Paul, you must take the right action. You must be physically active. Don't sit on a chair or sofa all day long. Move around. Do chores. Take a walk. Exercise!

How did I manage to lose 200 pounds in three to four months?

With exercise. That's what speeded up my weight loss. I started by walking up a steep hill. I walked less than one hundred yards on my first day. I walked real slow. I had to stop every couple of steps. But I went back every day. I walked more every day. Then I started walking faster. Four weeks later, I ran for a short time on the flat and downhill parts of the hill. Before I knew it, I was running uphill. That's when the fat melted off.

The Diet of Daniel only works if you exercise. Paul's mission only worked when he was physically active. That's why he took that first step on his travels. And he kept walking.

Think about Jesus. He was physically active. He walked all the time. To preach. To heal. To perform miracles.

Abraham walked to the Promised Land. Moses walked to freedom from Egypt. So did his people.

Be physically active. Abraham was active. Moses was active. Jesus was active. So was Paul. You too!

YOUR CHECKLIST FOR DAY 9

Right Thinking:

I work for my health. I am active. I exercise.

Right Eating:

- I eat the right foods in any amount. I do not go hungry. I do not eat sugar, bread, flour, or red meat. I eat lots of vegetables. If I must have meat, I eat fish or fowl (chicken, etc.).

- I drink plenty of water, alone or in herbal tea. I only drink pure water.

- I take a multi-vitamin, multi-mineral supplement. I also take fresh ginger root, selenium, and other supplements recommended by Dr. Andrew Weil, M.D.

Right Activity:

- I walk around the block for at least 25 minutes. Or swim. Or do another exercise.

- I read the Bible and pray for 15 minutes.

- I only snack on fresh vegetables or fruits.

- I am always active. I never sit down for more than 30 minutes.

THOUGHTS FOR DAY 9

RUN TO WIN!

> *You know that many runners enter a race, and only one of them wins the prize. So run to win!*
> —1 Corinthians 9:24, *CEV*

Life is like a race. You must: ***run to win!***

It's easy to start exercising. But you need to keep exercising on a regular basis. That's the key to success. Gyms have millions of dues-paying members. But more than half of all Americans are obese.

You won't lose weight or get healthy and fit if you are physically inactive.

It's true. *An idle soul shall suffer hunger* (Proverbs 19:15, *KJV*). You will think very little about eating if you are physically active. Get a hobby. Do chores. Just don't sit around and eat all the time.

Guess what happens when you're too busy to be hungry?

You eat less. You lose weight. You get fit. And when you eat, you eat the right foods.

PRACTICAL TIPS

What exercise should you do?

One that's right for your age and condition.

Are you 65? With mild arthritis? Try water aerobics. Or golf. Or another low-impact sport such as yoga.

Are you 40? And overweight? Walk. Keep walking until you can walk very fast. Then try running. Make sure your doctor says it's okay to do this.

Don't over do it. That'll get you sore. That usually becomes an excuse to stop exercising.

Try to exercise three times a week. That's the minimum. I sometimes exercise every day. Sometimes I just exercise three times a week.

Aerobic exercise is the best. That's where you sweat and breathe heavily for more than 15 minutes. Aerobic exercise burns fat. Your heart and lungs get stronger.

Your goal: 30 to 40 minutes of exercise.

10

RIGHT ACTIVITY

✦

DAY TEN: Choose The Right Activity

o o o o o o o o o o o o o o o o o o o o o o o o o o o o o o
Choose today whom you will serve…But as for me and my
family, we will serve the LORD.
—*Joshua 24:15, NLT*

I t's the last of the ten days. You've been tested for nine days. You've stuck to the diet. Great!

Daniel stuck to his diet for ten days. He could have dropped the diet at any time during the ten days. That would've been a very easy choice for Daniel. He could've chosen to be pampered with good food for the three years. He could've chosen to grow fat. And lazy.

Daniel had a good excuse for not going on his diet. Or for dropping out of the diet.

The excuse?

The order of a powerful king. Remember, the king ordered his servants to feed Daniel "a portion" of the king's meat and wine for three years (Daniel 1:5).

The king's food was extremely tempting. Back then, most people lived on meager diets. They ate very little. Two meals a day were a luxury. The best food was found in the king's palace. He was the wealthiest man of the land. That's why the best fed and the healthiest people were members of the royal family or those who worked for the king.

The king's food obviously appealed to Daniel. It appealed to his desires. And his appetites. Like Daniel, you're tempted with very appealing food. It appeals to your desires. And appetites.

But Daniel refused the king's "delicacies" and drink (Daniel 1:13, *NIV*).

Why?

Because Daniel knew that the king's refined foods and drinks would defile him. Daniel wanted to stay pure in body. And mind.

So Daniel went on his ten day diet. So have you!

In the end, Daniel won. He was healthy after the ten days. The king's servants saw that. They let him keep the diet for the rest of his life.

You know what happened when Daniel kept the diet the rest of his life. He prospered. He survived the lions' den. Kings respected him. He was a faithful servant of the Lord. Daniel was truly blessed.

Why did good things happen to Daniel?

Because he chose to honor God with his diet. So can you. Daniel stayed with the diet all his life. You can too.

But it all depends on your choices. Choose to think right about the diet and your health. Choose to eat right. Choose the right physical activities.

Show God that you're making the right choices. He will then bless you with long life and salvation. *With long life will I satisfy him and show him my salvation* (Psalms 91:16, *NIV*).

YOUR CHECKLIST FOR DAY 10

Right Thinking:

I choose to serve the LORD today. And every day. I eat right. And exercise right. I satisfy Him with long life. And show Him my salvation.

Right Eating:

- I eat the right foods in any amount. I do not go hungry. I do not eat sugar, bread, flour, or red meat. I eat lots of vegetables. If I must have meat, I eat fish or fowl (chicken, etc.).

- I drink plenty of water, alone or in herbal tea. I only drink pure water.

- I take a multi-vitamin, multi-mineral supplement. I also take fresh ginger root, selenium, and other supplements recommended by Dr. Andrew Weil, M.D.

Right Activity:

- I walk around the block for at least 30 minutes. Or swim. Or do another exercise.

- I read the Bible and pray for 15 minutes.

- I only snack on fresh vegetables or fruits.

- I am always active. I never sit down for more than 30 minutes.

THOUGHTS FOR DAY 10

GOOD AND BAD CARBS

Nature makes good carbohydrates. Vegetables have good carbs. So do fruits and grains. You easily digest good carbs. Your body's insulin metabolizes them in a snap. Good carbs give you energy. They do not make you fat.

It's bad carbs that make you fat.

Why?

Because they are concentrated. They've been processed and refined. They're like an atom bomb.

Where do you eat bad carbs?

In processed foods. And junk food. And fast food.

Want an example of a bad carb?

Sugar. It's everywhere. You'll find it mixed into most foods and drinks. Sometimes it's called "corn syrup". Other times it's called "fructose" or "dextrose".

Do you want to get really fat?

Then eat anything with flour.

It's true. Flour makes you fat. Flour makes you even fatter when you mix it with fat and/or sugar. Like bread. Cookies. Crackers. Most snack foods. Pizza. Almost all fast foods.

Flour comes from grain. But the grain has been milled or processed into a concentrated form. Flour makes you very fat unless you do tons of exercise.

TRUTH AND CONSEQUENCES

What happens when you eat bad carbs?

Your body makes too much insulin. Your fat cells then refuse to burn fat. You feel hungry all the time. That's how the extra insulin makes you fat.

Dr. Robert Atkins, M.D., knows all about "bad carbs". He explains them in his bestselling book: *Dr. Atkins' New Diet Revolution*.

TO START

I started my diet with the Dr. Atkins diet. The diet lets you lose lots of weight quickly. I did.

The Atkins diet is high in protein and fat. It has almost zero carbohydrates.

Go on the Atkins diet if you have to lose 100 or more pounds. After you lose the weight, switch to the Diet of Daniel. I did. Daniel's diet is far healthier. And it's kept my weight down for more than six years.

BALANCING YOUR WEIGHT

Your weight will go up and down over the years. That's natural. Your metabolism changes as you get older.

If you gain weight, then just do more exercise. Make sure you stick to the diet.

My weight went up two times.

I gained 15 pounds the first time. That was 10 years after I lost the 200 pounds.

How did I gain 15 pounds?

I got lazy. And stopped exercising. I was under a lot of stress at work. I started drinking a little whiskey. I did it to make sure I could fall asleep at night. Suddenly I couldn't fit into my pants. But I lost the 15 pounds easily. I started exercising again. And I never drank any alcohol again. I also made sure that I stopped eating bread. The 15 pounds were gone in two or three weeks.

I gained 30 pounds the second time. That was nine years after I lost the 15 pounds. I got lazy again. I stopped exercising. Sometimes I ate bread and other fattening foods.

I lost the 30 pounds easily. I started an intense exercise program of running up a steep hill. The 30 pounds were gone in four weeks. I lost so much weight that I had to double my calorie intake.

So don't panic as your weight goes up and down. Balance your weight with more exercise. Avoid bad carbs like the plague. It's been more than 20 years since I've had any fast food.

The secret to keeping to your ideal weight gain: right activity. Exercise! There are no shortcuts to good health and fitness.

Conclusions

It's up to you to be healthy. Trim. And fit.

Your health is in your hands. Sure, genetics and other factors play a role. But for the most part, it's up to you to be healthy, trim, and fit.

The 80-20 rule applies to your health and fitness. I say this based on my observations of other people as well as my own personal experiences.

Here's the rule: 80% of your health depends on what you eat; and, 20% depends on how much you exercise.

It's true. Food is so very important. It was right from the very beginning. Back to the Garden of Eden. Right after God made Adam and Eve.

Do you remember which food?

The fruit from the tree of good and evil.

God told Adam and Eve not to eat fruit from that tree (Genesis 3:2). But Eve was tempted by Satan. He told her to eat the fruit.

Do you remember what happened next?

The woman stared at the fruit. It looked beautiful and tasty (Genesis 3:6, *CEV*).

Eve then ate the fruit. She caved into temptation. So did Adam. They made a choice. It had eternal consequences. Mankind's future was changed forever.

God sent Adam and Eve out of the Garden of Eden (Genesis 3:23-24). Mankind now had to work for food. Death became part of life.

There are consequences to your choices.

So choose to eat right! And exercise! Good health and blessings will then come your way. Just like Daniel.

About the Author

Ernest Edsel, J.D., is the founder of Fitness Ministries. F.M. promotes Bible-based health and fitness. Ernest is a dynamic speaker. He has lectured at: leading corporations, law firms, and graduate schools. Ernest lives in Portland, Oregon. Visit Fitness Ministries at **www. intertruth.com**.

Appendix A

RIGHT LIVING

RIGHT SUPPLEMENTS

Take a ***multi-vitamin, multi-mineral supplement*** for adults. It must, at the very least, provide 100% of the daily recommended values for vitamins.

Try to take all your supplements with food.

Doctors and nutrition experts recommend ***40 grams of fiber*** a day. Most people take 20 grams or less. Take prunes or prune juice to make sure you get the fiber. Begin with two to four pitted prunes a day (more if not pitted). Or drink 1/4 cup of prune juice a day. Adjust as necessary.

Dr. Andrew Weil, M.D., recommends six more supplements in his book *8 Weeks to Optimum Health*.

1. ***Fresh ginger root.*** Take it as a tea or food. I put a few slices of fresh ginger root into a glass of water. I refill the glass with water throughout the day and drink the juice. Ginger is a great gastrointestinal and circulatory tonic.

2. ***Vitamin C,*** 2 to 6 grams per day. Take 1 to 3 grams (1,000-3,000 milligrams) two times a day, 12 hours apart. Only buy vitamin C with "rose hips". Do NOT buy chewable vitamin C.

3. ***Beta-carotene,*** 25,000 IU (international units) with breakfast. Only buy the *" **natural D. salina** "* formula. This formula gives you alpha-carotene, lutein, and zeaxanthin. They are very impor-

tant for your health. Lutein is for healthy eyes. Beta-carotene is a precursor of vitamin A. It's also an antioxidant, which prevents many diseases.

4. ***Vitamin E.*** Take 400 IU a day if you are less than 40 years old. Take 800 IU a day if you are more than 40 years old. Only buy the *"natural d-alpha"* formula. Do NOT buy the "dl-alpha" or other formula. Vitamin E is an anti-oxidant.

5. ***Selenium,*** 200 micrograms a day. Selenium is an anti-cancer trace mineral. Do NOT take it with your vitamin C. Selenium and vitamin C block each other. STOP taking selenium if you get peeling skin or fingernails or hair loss.

6. ***Aspirin,*** 80 to 162 milligrams a day. It prevents blood clots, which lead to heart attacks and strokes. Buy the cheapest aspirin. It's usually sold in standard 325 milligram (5 grain) pills. Cut these pills in half or in quarters.

RIGHT DRINKS

Drink water CONSTANTLY throughout the day in large amounts. Drink it alone. Or as an herbal tea (such as Stash). Most people don't drink enough water. They're dehydrated. That makes them feel hungry.

Reduce your hunger by drinking lots of water. And other zero or low calorie fluids.

If possible, ONLY drink carbon-filtered water or bottled spring water.

Avoid municipal water. It's full of chlorine (bleach) and/or flouride (a known carcinogen).

Cut back and eventually eliminate your intake of caffeine. Caffeine stimulates the release of insulin. Just like sugar. You get fatter or stay fat when your body makes lots of insulin. Caffeine also makes you nervous, even irritable.

If you can't stop drinking caffeine, then switch to green teas. They have polyphenols and catechins. These lower your cholesterol and improve lipid metabolism.

"Bad" drinks with caffeine include: coffee; teas that are made from dark or black tea leaves; and, almost all brands of soda pop.

I sweeten my herbal teas with fake sugar (Sweet and Lo). I'd rather not have the chemicals found in artificial sweeteners. But it's a trade off with obesity and all of its problems.

So if you want to lose weight or keep it down, then have lots of liquids all day long.

"Good" drinks or fluids include:

1. club soda;

2. essence flavored seltzer water ("no calories" must be on the label);

3. decaffeinated coffee or tea;

4. clear broth or bouillon soup (carefully read the label to make sure that the powder has no sugar or other carbs);

5. diet soda (preferably "caffeine-free");

6. iced tea with artificial sweetener;

7. lemon or lime juice (but note that it has almost 3 grams of carbohydrate per ounce).

Avoid grain beverages like imitation coffee made of barley. They have too many carbs.

Avoid alcoholic beverages. This means NO wine, beer, hard liquor, etc. You'll save your liver. And keep the pounds off.

RIGHT FOODS FOR WEIGHT LOSS

If you have to lose a lot of weight (more than 100 pounds), then the Dr. Atkins diet is for you. It's the only diet that really works. It sure worked for me! Read *Dr. Atkins' New Diet Revolution* by Robert C. Atkins, M.D. (1999 Avon Books).

Here's the Atkins diet in a nutshell:

1. Never have more than 20 grams of carbohydrates a day. This is equal to 3 cups of salad vegetables (loosely packed) or 2 cups of salad with 2/3 cup of cooked vegetables that have less than 10% carbohydrates (see list of low carb veggies in Day Eight).

2. Eat whenever you are hungry: it's the *type* of food that matters, not the quantity.

3. Eat any amount of protein. This means:

    a. any meat (lean beef, pork, lamb, veal, venison)

    b. any fish (flounder, salmon, trout, tuna, etc.);

    c. any shellfish (shrimp, lobster, crab, oysters, mussels, clams, squid, etc.);

    d. any fowl (chicken, goose, turkey, duck, cornish hen, quail, pheasant, etc.);

    e. any egg, cooked in any manner.

4. Have any amount of fat. This includes any amount of:

    a. butter, margarine, olive oil, mayonnaise, and cooking oil;

    b. any cheese (cheddar, mozzarella, swiss, cream cheese, cottage cheese, etc.), whether aged or fresh, cow or goat, hard or soft.

5. No diet cheese, cheese spreads, or whey cheeses. No imitation cheese products except for tofu (a soy cheese, but some brands add too many carbohydrates).

6. Do NOT eat carbohydrates! This means NO milk. No yogurt. No ice cream. NO bread. No cookies. No candy. No crackers.

7. Do NOT eat any carb combination such as carbohydrates with fat, carbohydrates with protein, carbohydrates with fat and protein.

8. Make sure NO SUGAR is added to any ingredient. Read your food's ingredients! Don't eat too many cold cuts since most have sugar (dextrose, etc.) and chemical preservatives. Stay away from processed meat products that are not 100% meat, fish, or fowl, such as imitation fish, meatloaf, and breaded foods.

A WORD ABOUT FATS AND OILS

God put the right amount of fat in grains, fruits, nuts, and vegetables. Avocados and salmon have healthy fats. Our bodies need some fats. Your cell walls are mostly made of fats (lipids). Your hormones are made of fats. Research shows that omega-3 oils are good for your heart. Healthy fats include gamma linolenic acid (GLA) and omega-3 oils. They are found in salmon and in linseed oil.

Olive oil is the healthiest oil. Other good oils are canola, walnut, soybean, sesame, sunflower, and safflower oils, especially if they are labeled "cold pressed."

Avoid "trans" oils and fats. They have trans-fatty acids, which are bad for your heart. "Trans" oils and fats include polyunsaturated vegetable oils, margarine, vegetable shortening, and all partially hydrogenated oils.

Deep-fried foods are loaded with bad "trans" oils. They are artery-cloggers. These oils are used to cook almost all snack foods. Like potato chips.

Butter is sometimes better than margarine. Many margarines have artery-clogging fats. Read the labels and compare, especially for the amount of saturated fats.

Watch out for coconut oil. It's pure poison for your heart.

Fast food companies always use artery-clogging fats. McDonald's, Burger King, Wendy's, Jack in the Box, and other fast food places will never use healthy oils or fats. They sure don't use oil and fat in small amounts.

PRACTICAL TIPS

Avoid beef and pork. They're full of bad fats. They'll clog your arteries.

Also consider this: cement, sawdust, and other fillers are regularly added to cattle feed. That information comes from television news shows like ABC's *20/20* and NBC's *Dateline*.

The less meat you eat, the better. Consider eggs. They're a great source of protein. They are not cholesterol bombs if boiled. Or cooked with a little olive oil.

GOOD FOODS

Check out **www.drweil.com**. It's the website of Dr. Weil, M.D. Go to the "Balanced Living" section. You will find great recipes. It also has lists of good and bad foods.

BUYER BEWARE

Always read the ingredient label. Read it before you buy the food or drink. Read it at home. Read it to avoid food loaded with sugar and other junk.

Make sure that NO sugar is added. Sugar includes dextrose and corn syrup.

Even canned tomatoes have added sugar!

So read the labels. Choose foods and drinks without any added sugar.

Avoid cold cuts. They're loaded with chemicals (nitrates). And lots of sugar (dextrose).

Avoid milk as much as possible.

Why?

Because milk is loaded with sugar (carbohydrates).

Don't believe me?

Read the label.

Don't get me wrong. The sugar isn't added to the milk. It's part of the cow's milk. But it's sugar. 100% fattening.

Even low-fat and no-fat ("skim") milk has sugar.

If you have to drink milk, then have soy milk or a low-fat organic milk.

Why?

Because it's the only way to avoid drinking Bovine Growth Hormone ("BGH").

BGH is injected into cows. It makes them produce huge amounts of milk.

What will BGH produce in your body when you drink it?

The FDA says BGH is safe for humans. But this is the same agency that let smokers think tobacco was safe for decades.

Buyer beware!

GO ORGANIC

Buy organic foods and drinks whenever possible. Organic means the food or drink is free of bad stuff.

What bad stuff?

Insecticides. Herbicides. Hormones. Other toxic chemicals.

RIGHT ACTIVITY

Walk, jog, run, or do any sport at least 30 minutes three times a week.

Build up slowly to this level of activity. Make sure your doctor tells you it's okay to do it. You may have to pick a different exercise if you have heart disease, including high blood pressure. Or if you have a joint or bone disaese, such as arthritis.

After appropriate training (and warming up), do your exercise such that you spend 15 to 30 minutes in your Target Heart Rate Zone (THRZ).

THRZ is your maximum aerobic condition. This means you are burning the most calories and body fat you can burn. THRZ strengthens your heart and lungs.

THRZ is based on 65% to 75% of your Predicted Maximal Heart Rate (PMHR).

Here's how you determine your Predicted Maximal Heart Rate (PMHR):

1. if you are an inactive person (never or rarely do any exercise), then your PHMR is 220 minus your age

    [220 - ..... = ... x .65 = ... beats/minute];

2. if you are an active person, your PHMR is 205 minus your age

    [205 - ..... = ... x .65 = ... beats/minute].

For example, the PHMR for an inactive 40 year old male or female is 117 [220 - 40 = 180 x .65 = 117].

To calculate your heart rate: press a finger on your wrist or neck. Count the pulse for six seconds. Then multiply by 10 (or count the pulse for 15 seconds, then multiply by 4).

TO GYM OR NOT TO GYM

It's better to exercise in the outdoors. Your muscles work more. Especially if you walk or run.

Why?

Because your leg muscles work much harder against hard surfaces in the outdoors.

Gyms, on the other hand, have workout machines. They are too soft for your legs.

Take treadmills. You might as well walk or run on pillows.

Treadmills and bicycles are great if you are more than 50 years old. Or if have a medical condition. Like knee or hip arthritis.

Gyms are also good if you live in a very cold or hot place.

Stepmills and "stair master" machines will help you burn lots of calories. Same with rowing machines.

ALWAYS MEASURE INCHES, NOT POUNDS

If you need to lose weight, measure your waist. Get a tape measure. Put it where your pant belt goes around your waist. This is the only true way to measure weight loss over a period of time.

Why?

Because if you just go by pounds, then you include a lot of variable factors, like water gain or loss.

The rule of thumb: one inch equals 15 pounds.

RECOMMENDED READING

These excellent books are available at libraries and new or used in your favorite bookstore.

1. *Dr. Atkins' New Diet Revolution* by Dr. Robert Atkins. M.D. [a "must read" if you are more than 100 pounds overweight].

2. *The Carbohydrate Addict's Diet* by Dr. Rachael Heller, Ph.D., and Dr. Richard Heller, Ph.D. [Their diet is similar to the Atkins diet, but they allow carbs. This makes some people break the diet and give up. The book will help you understand why the foods in

Daniel's diet are so filling and why junk food and fast food make you hungry].

3. ***Eight Weeks to Optimum Health*** by Dr. Andrew Weil, M.D. [highly recommended; a "must read" if you want to be healthy].

4. ***The Pritikin Weight Loss Breakthrough*** by Robert Pritikin [highly recommended; a "must read". He believes in the Diet of Daniel. The book has excellent recipes for foods in Diet of Daniel]. Or, read *The Pritikin Program for Diet and Exercise* by Nathan Pritikin.]

5. *The Aerobics Program for Well-Being* by Dr. Kenneth Cooper, M.D. He also wrote *Aerobics*. [both books show why aerobic exercise is so important for good health and fitness].

APPENDIX B

FOUR SCIENTIFIC FACTS ABOUT THE DIET OF DANIEL

FACT #1: THE DIET PREVENTS CANCER

Research shows that 60 to 70% of all cancers can be prevented.

How?

Through simple changes in your diet and lifestyle. By eating healthy. Staying active. Watching your weight. And not drinking or smoking. That's how you substantially reduce your risk of cancer.

The source for this information: the American Institute for Cancer Research (**www.aicr.org**).

AICR is the nation's third largest cancer charity. It's also a pioneer in the role of diet and nutrition in the prevention and treatment of cancer.

FACT #2: YOU ARE WHAT YOU EAT (AND SMOKE)

Every year, half a million Americans die of cancer. Evidence suggests that diet is big factor in the 500,000 deaths.

How big a factor?

One-third. Yes, that big a factor. One third of the 500,000 deaths are due to diet.

Guess what's a factor for another 1/3 of the deaths?

Cigarette smoking.

The source for this information: the American Cancer Society. Doctors and experts believe in a healthy diet like the Diet of Daniel.

See the "Health Information Seekers" section in the Cancer Society's website (**www.cancer.org**).

FACT #3: FOREVER YOUNG

If you want to prevent heart disease, then keep the Diet of Daniel.

The American Heart Association recommends a diet like the Diet of Daniel. See the "Healthy Lifestyle" section in their website (**www.americanheart.org**).

Daniel's diet will help you lose weight. And it will help you control your diabetes. Just look at the "Healthy Living" section in the website of the American Diabetes Association (**www.diabetes.org**).

FACT #4: AMERICA NEEDS THE DIET OF DANIEL

The U.S. Surgeon General issued a troubling report on our eating and exercise habits. It's called "The Surgeon General's Call To Action To Prevent and Decrease Overweight and Obesity". The report is available at the U.S. Surgeon General's website (**www.surgeongeneral.gov/topics/obesity/**).

Here's an important section of the report:

"The total direct and indirect costs attributed to overweight and obesity amounted to $117 billion in the year 2000. In 1999, an estimated 61 percent of U.S. adults were overweight, along with 13 percent of children and adolescents.

"Obesity among adults has doubled since 1980, while overweight among adolescents has tripled.

"Only 3 percent of all Americans meet at least four of the five federal Food Guide Pyramid recommendations for the intake of grains, fruits, vegetables, dairy products, and meats.

"And less than one-third of Americans meet the federal recommendations to engage in at least 30 minutes of moderate physical activity at least five days a week, while 40 percent of adults engage in no leisure-time physical activity at all."

APPENDIX C

MY DIET JOURNAL

Use this journal to record: your waist measurement; and, the amount of time you spend on exercise. This is the best way to track how well you are following the Diet of Daniel.

I began the Diet of Daniel on the .... day of .... in the year ....

I. MY WAIST MEASUREMENT (in inches):

.... inches on day 1

.... inches on day 10

.... inches on day 20

.... inches on day 30 (first month; week 4)

Then take waist measurements every 2 weeks:

.... inches at week 6

.... inches at week 8 (second month)

.... inches at week 10

.... inches at week 12 (third month)

.... inches at week 14

.... inches at week 16 (fourth month)

.... inches at week 18

.... inches at week 20 (fifth month)

.... inches at week 22

.... inches at week 24 (sixth month

.... inches at week 26

.... inches at week 28 (seventh month)

.... inches at week 30

.... inches at week 32 (eighth month)

.... inches at week 34

.... inches at week 36 (ninth month)

.... inches at week 38

.... inches at week 40

.... inches at week 42 (tenth month)

.... inches at week 44

.... inches at week 46

.... inches at week 48 (eleventh month)

.... inches at week 50

.... inches at week 52 (twelfth month)

II. MY TIME SPENT ON EXERCISE (in minutes; this time does not include time spent warming up).

.... minutes on day 1 (try at least 15 min.)

.... minutes on day 2 (try at least 15 min.)

.... minutes on day 3 (try at least 15 min.)

.... minutes on day 4 (try at least 20 min.)

.... minutes on day 5 (try at least 20 min.)

.... minutes on day 6 (try at least 20 min.)

.... minutes on day 7 (try at least 25 min.)

.... minutes on day 8 (try at least 25 min.)

.... minutes on day 9 (try at least 25 min.)

.... minutes on day 10 (try at least 30 min.)

*After day 10, exercise for **at least 30 minutes every day** for the next 30 days.*

.... minutes on day 11

.... minutes on day 12

.... minutes on day 13

.... minutes on day 14

.... minutes on day 15

.... minutes on day 16

.... minutes on day 17

.... minutes on day 18

.... minutes on day 19

.... minutes on day 20

.... minutes on day 21

.... minutes on day 22

.... minutes on day 23

.... minutes on day 24

.... minutes on day 25

.... minutes on day 26

.... minutes on day 27

.... minutes on day 28

.... minutes on day 29

.... minutes on day 30

After day 30, make sure you exercise at least 30 minutes 3 times a week!

0-595-21812-1

Printed in the United States
56085LVS00007B/128